Comfortable Expectations: An Overview of Sitting and Sleeping Positions During Pregnancy
By

Claire L. Womack

Copyright :

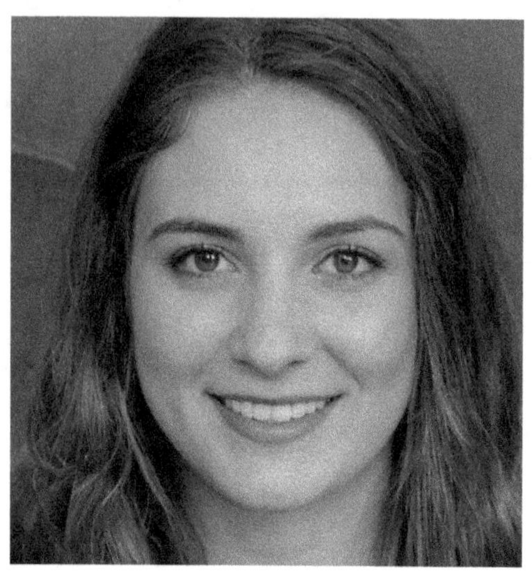

About the author

Claire L. Womack is a dedicated author with an establishment in nursing, focusing on giving presence of mind encounters to energetic mothers. Her work presumably spins around keeping an eye on the various pieces of pregnancy, offering bearing, and helping women with investigating the trip to life as a parent. By combining her nursing dominance excitedly for supporting energetic moms,Claire means to draw in women with significant information and resources during this unprecedented great time.

While expressing experiences concerning Claire L. Womack life and business could require a more start to finish assessment, her commitment to help excited mothers suggests a kind and taught approach. It's conceivable that her organizations jump into subjects like pre-birth care, work status, post-pregnancy success, and maybe even newborn child care.Claire likely draws from her nursing experience to offer confirmation based direction, empowering a sensation of sureness and availability for mothers to-be as they investigate the hardships and joys of pregnancy. For a total cognizance of her work, examining her conveyed books, articles, or any reasonable gatherings would give further pieces of information into her responsibilities to maternal prosperity.

Introduction

Certainly! Here is a drawing in presentation for "Comfortable Expectations]: An Outline of Sitting and sleeping Positions During Pregnancy" by Claire L. Womack

Congrats on this lovely excursion! " Comfortable Expectations digs into the nuanced specialty of sitting and sleeping positions during pregnancy, offering an adroit and supporting viewpoint on exploring the fundamental parts of Comfort and prosperity.

In this exhaustive aide, Claire L. Womack offers a profound plunge into the universe of maternal Comfort, introducing a variety of fundamental tips, systems, and master counsel custom-made to help eager people all through their pregnancy process.

From consoling experiences on ideal guest plans to encouraging tranquil and soothing evenings, "Comfortable Expectations fills in as a key sidekick, furnishing eager people with the information and devices to advance their prosperity as they get ready to invite their little one.

"Comfortable Expectations]" offers an incorporating look into the specialty of sitting and sleeping position during the extraordinary long stretches of pregnancy.

This acquaintance points with dazzle perusers, welcoming them into a universe of maternity Comfort and prosperity, as investigated by Claire L. Womack in her thorough aide.

Chapter 1

Embracing Comfort

Pregnancy is a surprising and groundbreaking experience, both genuinely and inwardly. It carries with it an outpouring of changes, and it's simply normal to need to guarantee the greatest possible level of Comfort for yourself during this period. Establishing a climate that takes care of your prosperity isn't just valuable for you yet additionally adds to the positive improvement of your developing child.

One of the most vital phases in embracing Comfort during pregnancy is to put resources into maternity clothing that fits well as well as causes you to feel sure and quiet. The progressions in your body can be both energizing and testing, and having clothing that adjusts to these progressions can have a tremendous effect. Indulge yourself with agreeable textures that permit your skin to inhale, and don't be hesitant to grandstand your special style through maternity design.

Focusing on rest is one more key part of embracing Comfort during pregnancy. Your body is working indefatigably to sustain and uphold the existence developing inside you. It's fundamental to pay attention to its signs and permit yourself the time you want to re-energize. Quality rest is a valuable product during pregnancy, so think about putting resources into steady pads and establishing a comfortable rest climate that energizes serene evenings.

Delicate activities, like pre-birth yoga, can likewise add to your general Comfort. In addition to the fact that it eases normal pregnancy distresses, however it likewise advances adaptability and unwinding. Participating in exercises that support your body and brain won't just upgrade your actual prosperity yet in addition set you up for the impending changes.

. Encircle yourself with things that give you pleasure and unwinding. Whether it's delicate covers, mitigating aromas, or quieting music, tailor your current circumstance to mirror the harmony and serenity you merit.

 the event that you wind up requiring help or backing, make sure to out. Surround yourself with companions, family, and medical care experts who grasp the significance of your Comfort

In embracing Comfort during pregnancy, you are supporting yourself as well as encouraging a positive and sustaining climate for your developing family into parenthood.

Chapter 2

Supporting maternal prosperity: Pregnancy and parenthood

Pregnancy is an extraordinary and euphoric time in a lady's life, however it can likewise achieve huge changes to her psychological wellness.

While many spotlight on the actual parts of pregnancy, it is pivotal not to ignore the profound prosperity of hopeful moms. Pregnancy can set off a scope of feelings, from fervor and joy to tension and emotional episodes.

Overview of Pregnancy

Pregnancy is joined by a hurricane of feelings. Hormonal vacillations, actual uneasiness, and the expectation of becoming a parent can prompt uplifted close to home responsiveness and emotional episodes. It is fundamental for eager moms to perceive that these profound changes are typical and to rehearse self-sympathy.

Keeping up with open lines of correspondence with medical care suppliers, accomplices, and friends and family can offer an important help organization. Sharing sentiments and concerns can mitigate uneasiness and assist with dealing with close to home prosperity. Participating in unwinding procedures, like profound breathing, reflection, or pre-birth yoga, can likewise advance close to home equilibrium and lessen feelings of anxiety.

Tension and Pregnancy-Related Stresses

Pregnancy frequently achieves increased nervousness and stress. Worries about the wellbeing and prosperity of the child, the birthing system, and the difficulties of parenthood can weigh intensely on eager moms' psyches. Unreasonable nervousness during pregnancy can prompt rest unsettling influences, expanded circulatory strain, and influence generally speaking maternal prosperity.

To address pregnancy-related stresses, it is significant for eager moms to look for help and dependable data. Building areas of strength for an organization that incorporates medical care experts, accomplices, family, and companions can give a feeling of consolation and direction. Taking part in labor schooling classes and pre-birth support gatherings can likewise offer significant assets and associations with other eager moms.

Selfcare during pregnancy

Rehearsing taking care of oneself is crucial during this time. Participating in exercises that advance unwinding, like scrubbing down, perusing, or appreciating delicate activity, can assist with diminishing nervousness levels.

Integrating pressure from the executives' strategies, like care or journaling, into day to day schedules can likewise give a feeling of quiet and advance mental prosperity.

Postpartum depression

Pregnancy and the post pregnancy time frame can likewise expand the gamble of perinatal state of mind issues, like pre-birth despondency and postpartum anxiety. These circumstances can essentially influence a mother's emotional wellness and her capacity to bond with and care for her child.

is fundamental for medical care suppliers and friends and family to be watchful for indications of perinatal state of mind problems and to offer proper help and assets. Standard pre-birth check-ups ought to incorporate psychological wellness screenings to distinguish potential worries from the get-go. Instruction and mindfulness about perinatal mind-set problems can assist with eliminating the disgrace encompassing them, making it more straightforward for ladies to look for help without judgement or disgrace.

Treatment choices for postpartum depression

issues might incorporate treatment, support gatherings, and, now and again, medicine. Teaming up with medical services experts and emotional well-being suppliers can guarantee an extensive and customized way to deal with overseeing perinatal psychological well-being.

Building Areas of strength

Building areas of strength is significant for hopeful and new moms to keep up with their psychological prosperity. Backing can emerge out of accomplices, relatives, companions, and medical care suppliers. A strong encouraging group of people gives a place of refuge to sharing worries, getting direction, and feeling approved in the excursion of motherhood.Partners can assume an essential part in supporting maternal emotional well-being. Taking part in open correspondence, effectively partaking in pre-birth arrangements, and offering close to home help can have a tremendous effect in the prosperity of hopeful and new moms. Loved ones can offer functional help, for example, assist with family tasks or child care, to lessen pressure and take into account taking care of oneself.

Furthermore, interfacing with other hopeful and new moms through help gatherings or online networks can give a feeling of fellowship and approval. Sharing encounters, looking for counsel, and getting support from ladies going through comparative circumstances can mitigate sensations of disengagement and upgrade mental prosperity

Pregnancy is a surprising excursion loaded up with fervor, challenges, and significant profound changes. Sustaining maternal mental prosperity during this extraordinary period is fundamental for the general wellbeing and bliss of both the mother and the child.

Chapter 3

Good Posture During Pregnancy

Posture is the situation where you hold your body while standing, sitting, or resting. Great posture during pregnancy includes preparing your body to stand, walk, sit, and lie in places where the least strain is put on your back.

Great posture (the situation wherein you hold your body while standing, sitting, or resting) during pregnancy includes preparing your body to stand, walk, sit, and lie in places where minimal strain is put on your back. In spite of the fact that your developing stomach might cause you to feel like you will be brought down, there are a few stages you can take to keep up with great posture and legitimate body mechanics. Here are a few hints.

Right Method for Standing During Pregnancy:

- Hold your head up straight with your jaw in. Try not to shift your head forward, in reverse, down, or sideways.

- Ensure your ear cartilage is in accordance with the centre of your shoulders.

- Position your shoulder bones back and move your chest forward.

- Keep your knees straight, yet not entirely locked.

- Stretch the highest point of your head toward the roof.

- Pull your stomach in and up (however much could be expected!). Try not to shift your pelvis forward or in reverse. Keep your bum wrapped up.

- Point your feet in a similar direction, with your weight adjusted uniformly between the two feet. The curves of your feet ought to be upheld with low-behaved (however not level) shoes to forestall weight on your back.

- Try not to remain similarly situated for quite a while.

- On the off chance that you really want to represent extensive stretches, change the level of the work table to an agreeable level if conceivable.

Attempt to lift one foot by laying it on a stool or box. After a few minutes, switch your foot position.

While working in the kitchen, open the cupboard under the sink and lay one foot within the cupboard but change foot after some minutes

How to sit in pregnancy:

- Keep awake with your back straight and your shoulders back. Your bum should contact the back of your seat.

- Sit with a back help (like a little, rolled-up towel or a lumbar roll) at the twist of your back. Pregnancy pads are sold at various retailers.

This is the method for finding a good sitting position when you're not using a back help or lumbar roll:

- Sit around the completion of your seat and slouch completely.

- Draw yourself up and supplement the twist of your back past what many would think about conceivable. Hold for two or three minutes.

- Release the position fairly (around 10 degrees). This is a nice sitting position.

- Flow your body weight fairly on the two hips.

- Keep your hips and knees at a right point (use a stool if fundamental). Your legs should not be crossed and your feet should be level on the floor.

Endeavour to do whatever it takes not to sit also arranged for north of 30 minutes.

At work, change your seat level and workstation so you can sit up close to your workspace. Rest your elbows and arms on your seat or workspace, keeping your shoulders free.

While sitting in a seat that rolls and turns, don't bend at the midsection while sitting. Taking everything into account, turn your whole body.

While standing up from the sitting position, move to the front of the seat. Stand up by fixing your legs. Make an effort not to wind forward at your waist. Subsequent to standing, do a couple of pregnancy-safeguarded back broadens.

It is okay to acknowledge other sitting circumstances for short periods of time, yet by far most of your sitting time should be spent as portrayed above so there is inconsequential load on your back. If you have back torture, sit as little as could truly be anticipated, and only for short periods of time.

Driving During Pregnancy:

Use a back help (lumbar roll) at the twist of your back while driving when pregnant. Your knees should be at a comparative level or higher than your hips.

Move the seat close to the directing wheel, yet at a similar not unreasonably close. When in doubt, your seat should be adequately near, grant your knees to contort and your feet to show up at the pedals. Your stomach should be something like 10 downers from the coordinating wheel, if possible (this plainly depends on your level). The last month of pregnancy, when your waist is most likely going to be closer than at some other opportunity to the coordinating wheel, ride in the explorer's seat at whatever point what is happening permits.

Constantly wear both the lap and shoulder seat lashes. Place the lap belt under your waist, as missing the mark on your hips as could truly be anticipated and across your upper thighs. Never place the belt over your mid-locale. Place the shoulder belt between your chests. Change the shoulder and lap belts as comfortable as could truly be anticipated.

Expecting that your vehicle is furnished with an air pack, it is imperative to wear your shoulder and lap belts. Furthermore, reliably sit back something like 10 inches away from the site where the air sack is taken care of. On the driver's side, the air sack is arranged in the directing wheel. While driving, pregnant women should change the directing wheel with the objective that it is inclined toward the chest and away from the head .

How to lift objects during pregnancy

- Demand help while lifting significant articles when you're pregnant.

- Before you lift an article, guarantee you have firm equilibrium.

- To get an article that is lower than the level of your midriff, keep your back straight and curve at your knees and hips. Make an effort not to curve forward at the waist with your knees straight.

- Stand with a wide situation close to the thing you are endeavouring to get and keep your feet firm on the ground. Fix your stomach muscles and lift the article using your leg muscles. Fix your knees in a reliable development. Make an effort not to yank the thing up to your body.

- Stand absolutely upstanding without distorting.

- Expecting you are lifting a thing from a table, slide it to the edge of the table so you can hold it close to your body.

Contort your knees so you are close to the article. Use your legs to lift the thing and come to a standing position.

- Utilize alert while lifting significant articles above midriff level.

- Hold packs close to your body with your arms bent. Keep your stomach muscles tight. Take little steps and go continuously.

- To cut down the article, place your feet as you did to lift, fix stomach muscles, and contort your hips and knees.Try to lean forward.

- While collecting something above:

- Guarantee you have a brilliant thought about how significant the thing is that you will lift.
- Use two hands to lift.

Chapter 4

Sleep during pregnancy

Why is sleep so important during pregnancy? Sleep is the point at which your body resets and fixes itself. It's the point at which your mind gains experiences, making it a partner in your fight against child cerebrum. It's the way your veins reestablish themselves, which is particularly significant now that they're under expanded strain from the additional blood stream expected to help your child.sleep likewise keeps your resistant framework — which is stifled to help your pregnancy — solid. Furthermore, sleep controls how your body responds to insulin; not obtaining an adequate number results in a higher glucose level, increasing your gamble of gestational diabetes.

Sleeping positions in pregnancy:

Sleeping on your back during pregnancy

A few specialists suggest pregnant ladies abstain from dozing on their backs during the second and third trimesters. Why? The back rest position rests the whole weight of the developing uterus and child on your back, your digestive organs and your vena cava, the primary vein that conveys blood to your heart.

Previously, the idea was that lying on your side upgraded blood return to your heart and in this manner advanced oxygenated blood getting to your child. Yet, a few specialists currently express that there's no genuine distinction in results to children of mother's who rest negligible time on their back or more often than not of their back.

Sleeping to your left side or right side during pregnancy

During the second and third trimesters, dozing on one or the other side — ideally the left, if conceivable — is viewed by certain specialists to be great for yourself as well as your child-to-be.

This position considers greatest blood stream and supplements to the placenta (and that implies less strain on the vena cava) and upgrades kidney capability, and that implies better end of side-effects and less enlarging in your feet, lower legs and hands.

Tips on comfortable pregnancy sleeping positions

Get a remarkable cushion. For extra assistance, make a pass at using a wedge-shaped cushion or a 5-foot full-body pregnancy cushion.

Set yourself up. If pads don't help, make a pass at resting in a semi-upstanding circumstance in a seat (expecting you have one) as opposed to the bed.

Keep in mind, it's not surprising to feel abnormal for two or three nights or even a portion of a month. Your body will surely adjust to another position given time.

Envision a situation in which you stir laying on your back in pregnancy.

Relatively few people stay there in their psyche throughout the span of the night. If you stir while laying on your back during pregnancy, or on your stomach, you can unwind (repeat: just take it easy). No harm done.

Yet again the way that you stirred regardless is in all probability your pregnant body's way to deal with encouraging you to change positions (and maybe go to the washroom, another ordinary pregnancy rest issue).

Isn't getting adequate rest destructive to me or my youngster?

By a wide margin the majority of women truth be told do encounter some trouble resting, so take the necessary steps not to push if you're not getting as many areas of strength for much eye as you were pre-pregnancy. In light of everything, research has shown that women who relentlessly hit the sack for under six hours a night could have longer works and will undoubtedly require C-fragments.

Untreated rest apnea, where breathing is vexed generally throughout the span of the late night inciting awful rest and late night waking, has been associated with pregnancy burdens including pre-eclampsia, gestational hypertension and low birth weight. Accepting that you figure you could encounter the evil impacts of this condition, make sure to chat with your PCP.

Unsure of accepting at least for now that you're getting the ideal extent of rest? The best method for making a decision isn't by how long you clock in lying in bed yet by how you feel. In case you track down that you're not snoozing and are tenaciously depleted — past the average weariness of pregnancy — you're not getting adequate rest.

Accepting that you consider need rest is transforming into an issue, banter with your clinical benefits proficient. The individual can help you with finding the underpinning of your anxiety and deals with serious consequences regarding getting the rest you truly care about.

Experts have commonly said that the best rest position while you're expecting is on your left side — anyway your right is furthermore completely alright. Past your most significant trimester, it becomes hard to lie on your stomach for clear reasons.

Various experts in like manner propose that you do whatever it takes not to lie level on your back the whole night. Regardless, a couple of experts as of now say that pregnant moms can remain in bed any spot that is pleasing for them rather than stress significantly done with everything some way or another.

Overall, pregnant women should really try not to lie level on their back or clearly on their stomach. Lying on your back, especially in the third trimester, causes more work and weight on your heart: Here, the youngster's weight can descend on the below average vena cava, the gigantic vein that conveys blood from the feet and legs, pelvis, and mid-district back to the heart, lessening circulatory system to the placenta. Moreover, laying on your back can truly cause you to have a spinal aggravation!

Lying on your stomach during pregnancy isn't likely going to be really pleasant. Even more essentially, lying on your stomach should be avoided considering the way that it can descend on the undeveloped organism and reduce circulation.

Make an effort not to be unnecessarily concerned about expecting you to shift positions at night; this is a regular piece of snoozing that you have zero command over. Probably, expecting that you end up lying on your back or stomach, the trouble will stir you.

A couple of experts recommend that pregnant women lie on their given side in the third trimester to consider the best circulation system to the child, uterus and kidneys. Since your liver is on the right 50% of your body, lying on the left side moreover helps keep the uterus away from pushing on that gigantic organ.

Despite what position you lie in, a pad should be under your head, but not your shoulders, and should be a thickness that allows your head to be in a standard circumstance to make an effort not to strain your back. You may in like manner need to put a cushion between your legs for help. Use your pads to find an open to resting position. A couple phenomenal "pregnancy" pads are sold that may be valuable to you to rest better.

Endeavour to rest in a spot that helps you with staying aware of the curve in your back, (for instance, on your side with your knees to some degree bowed and with a cushion between your knees). Do whatever it takes not to lay on your side with your knees pulled in up to your chest.

Select a strong sheet material and box spring set that doesn't list. In the event that principal, place a board under your bedding. You can in like manner put the dozing pad on the floor for a short time frame if fundamental.

If you have reliably napped on a sensitive surface, it may be more challenging to change to a hard surface. Endeavour to do what is by and large pleasing for you.

While standing up from the lying position, happen to your side, draw up the two knees and swing your legs to the bed's side. Sit up by driving yourself up with your hands. Do whatever it takes not to curve forward at your midriff

Why Does Pregnancy Sometimes Make Sleeping Difficult?

Exactly when you're pregnant, getting a fair night's rest can be hard. As you get more prominent, it gets more enthusiastic to find a content resting position. You would need to pee around 12 PM. Besides, indigestion can stir you.

A couple of women have leg issues and spinal torments, especially as they begin conveying progressively more weight. Various pregnant women report that their dreams become surprisingly clear, and some even have terrible dreams.

Stress can hinder rest too. Maybe you're worried about your kid's prosperity, fretful about your abilities as a parent, or having a restless point of view toward genuine transport. This huge number of opinions are average, but they could keep you (and your associate) up around night time.

How Should I Get a Prevalent Night's Rest?

From the outset in your pregnancy, endeavour to begin snoozing on your side. Lying on your side with your knees contorted is presumably going to be the most pleasing circumstance as your pregnancy progresses. It moreover simplifies your heart's occupation because it keeps the kid's weight away from applying strain to the gigantic vein (called the average vena cava) that passes blood back on to the heart from your feet and legs.

Regardless, don't make yourself crazy by focusing on what you could turn over onto your back during the night. Moving positions is a trademark piece of napping that you have zero command over.

Have a go at attempting various things with cushions to find an open to snoozing position. A couple of women place a pad under their mid-locale or between their legs. Similarly, using a bunched up cushion or rolled-up cover at the tad of your back could help with facilitating some strain. In all honesty, you'll see a seriously enormous number of "pregnancy pads" accessible. If you're contemplating getting one, talk with your essential consideration doctor first about which could work for you.

Over-the-counter sedatives, including local fixes, are not recommended for pregnant women.

Tips for getting a good night sleep:

Eliminate invigorated drinks like pop, coffee, and tea from your eating routine whatever amount as could be anticipated. Limit any confirmation of them to the morning or afternoon.

Go without drinking a lot of fluids or eating a full banquet inside two or three significant lengths of stirring things up around town. (Regardless, guarantee that you in like manner get a great deal of enhancements and liquids throughout the day.) A couple of women find it strong to have more at breakfast and lunch and a while later have a more unassuming dinner. If disorder keeps you up, make a pass at eating two or three wafers before you hit the sack.

Get into a day to day timetable of making a beeline for rest and arousing all the while each day.

Avoid exhaustive action not long before you hit the sack. In light of everything, achieve something loosening up, like examining a book or having a warm, sans caffeine drink, similar to draining it with honey or some regular tea.

In case a leg cramp mixes you, it could help with pressing your feet hard against the wall or to stay on the leg. A couple of women find that expanding their lower leg muscles before bed has an effect. Similarly, guarantee that you're getting adequate calcium and magnesium in your eating schedule, which can help with diminishing leg cramps. However, take no upgrades without checking with your PCP.

Take a yoga class or learn other loosening up strategies to help you with relaxing following a clamouring day. (Make sure to inspect any new development or wellbeing routine with your essential doctor first.)

If fear and disquiet are keeping you cognizant, consider pursuing a work class or sustaining class. More data and the association of other pregnant women could help with working with the sensations of fear that keep you alert around night time.

Think about how conceivable it is that I Really Can't Rest.

Clearly, there will be times when you can't rest. As opposed to flailing wildly, focusing on that you're not resting, and counting the hours until your morning clock will go off, get up and achieve something hing calm: read a book, focus on music, or look at a magazine. Eventually, you'll probably feel drained enough to get back to rest.

In addition, if possible, set down for brief reprieves (30 60 minutes) during on the day. Rests can help you with having energy to conquer the day and give your body the rest it needs.

Conclusion

As we close the last shade on "Agreeable Assumptions: An Outline of Sitting and Dozing Positions During Pregnancy" by Claire L. Womack, it is our sincerest desire that this savvy guide has offered direction, yet additionally bestowed a feeling of serene confirmation in the midst of the groundbreaking phases of pregnancy.

May the insight and supporting experiences shared inside these pages keep on being an unfaltering sidekick, offering solace, consolation, and imperativeness fundamental for this striking period of life.

Explore the peaceful specialty of seating and lay down with the recently discovered information and supporting direction presented inside these parts. May the solace and prosperity procedures spread out by Claire L. Womack act as delicate partners on your amazing excursion, cultivating quiet, peacefulness, and the imperativeness fundamental for this lovely period of life.

Embrace every second with a feeling of consolation, knowing that "Agreeable Assumptions" remains as a supporting reference point, offering a loved hug to direct you through each great assumption for pregnancy.

Here's to an excursion loaded up with solace, satisfaction, and the peaceful consolation that each second is an esteemed one.

As you set out on the wondrous excursion ahead, recollect that sustaining solace isn't simply an assumption; It is an exquisitely deserved fact.

Congrats on this noteworthy excursion!